The New Selection of Plant Based Diet Recipes

50 Innovative Dishes for your Diet

Joanna Vinson

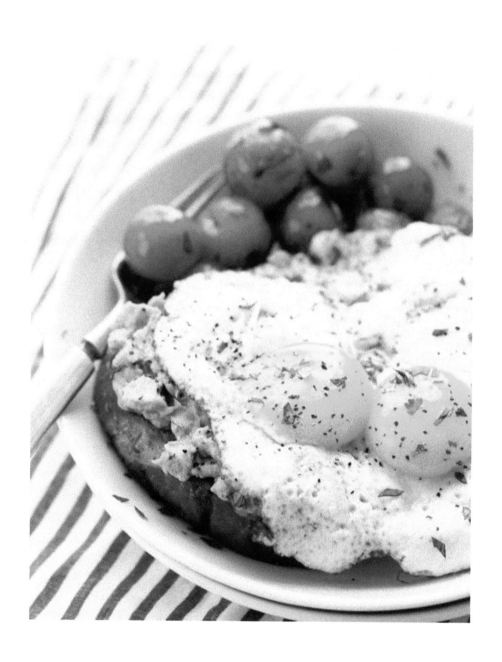

TABLE OF CONTENTS

Carrot and Chocolate Bread

Preparation Time: 5-15 minutes | Cooking Time: 75 minutes | Servings: 4

Ingredients:

For the dry mix:

- 1 ½ cup whole-wheat flour
- ¼ cup almond flour
- ¼ tsp salt
- ¼ tsp cloves powder
- ¼ tsp cayenne pepper
- 1 tbsp cinnamon powder
- ½ tsp nutmeg powder
- ½ tsp baking soda
- 1 ½ tsp baking powder

For the wet batter:

- 2 tbsp flax seed powder + 6 tbsp water
- ½ cup pure date sugar
- ¼ cup pure maple syrup
- ¾ tsp almond extract
- 1 tbsp grated lemon zest
- ½ cup unsweetened applesauce

- ¼ cup olive oil

- **For folding into the batter**:

- 4 carrots, shredded
- 3 tbsp unsweetened chocolate chips
- 2/3 cup black raisins

Directions:

1. Preheat the oven to 375 F and line an 8x4 loaf tin with baking paper.
2. In a large bowl, mix all the flours, salt, cloves powder, cayenne pepper, cinnamon powder, nutmeg powder, baking soda, and baking powder.
3. In another bowl, mix the flaxseed powder, water, and allow thickening for 5 minutes. Mix in the date sugar, maple syrup, almond extract, lemon zest, applesauce, and olive oil.
4. Combine both mixtures until smooth and fold in the carrots, chocolate chips, and raisins.
5. Pour the mixture into a loaf pan and bake in the oven until golden brown on top or a toothpick inserted into the bread comes out clean, 45 to 60 minutes.
6. Remove from the oven, transfer the bread onto a wire rack to cool, slice, and serve.

Nutrition:

Calories 524 | Fats 15. 8g | Carbs 94. 3g | Protein 7. 9g

Pineapple French Toasts

Preparation Time: 5-15 minutes | Cooking Time: 55 minutes | Servings: 4

Ingredients:

- 2 tbsp flax seed powder + 6 tbsp water
- 1 ½ cups unsweetened almond milk
- ½ cup almond flour
- 2 tbsp pure maple syrup + extra for drizzling
- 2 pinches salt
- ½ tbsp cinnamon powder
- ½ tsp fresh lemon zest
- 1 tbsp fresh pineapple juice
- 8 whole-grain bread slices

Directions:

1. Preheat the oven to 400 F and lightly grease a roasting rack with olive oil.
2. Set aside.
3. In a medium bowl, mix the flax seed powder with water and allow thickening for 5 to 10 minutes.

4. Whisk in the almond milk, almond flour, maple syrup, salt, cinnamon powder, lemon zest, and pineapple juice.

5. Soak the bread on both sides in the almond milk mixture and allow sitting on a plate for 2 to 3 minutes.

6. Heat a large skillet over medium heat and place the bread in the pan. Cook until golden brown on the bottom side. Flip the bread and cook further until golden brown on the other side, 4 minutes in total.

7. Transfer to a plate, drizzle some maple syrup on top and serve immediately.

Nutrition:

Calories 294 | Fats 4. 7g |Carbs 52. 0g | Protein 11. 6g

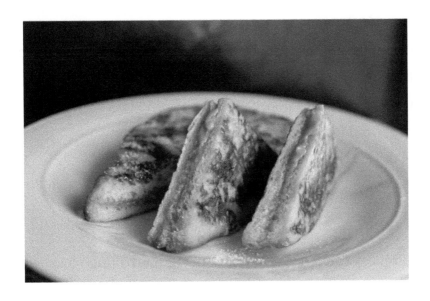

Pimiento Cheese Breakfast Biscuits

Preparation Time: 5-15 minutes | Cooking Time: 30 minutes | Servings: 4

Ingredients:

- 2 cups whole-wheat flour
- 2 tsp baking powder
- 1 tsp salt
- ½ tsp baking soda
- ½ tsp garlic powder
- ¼ tsp black pepper
- ¼ cup unsalted plant butter, cold and cut into 1/2-inch cubes
- ¾ cup of coconut milk
- 1 cup shredded cashew cheese
- 1 (4 oz) jar chopped pimientos, well-drained
- 1 tbsp melted unsalted plant butter

Directions:

1. Preheat the oven to 450 F and line a baking sheet with parchment paper.
2. Set aside.

3. In a medium bowl, mix the flour, baking powder, salt, baking soda, garlic powder, and black pepper.
4. Add the cold butter using a hand mixer until the mixture is the size of small peas.
5. Pour in ¾ of the coconut milk and continue whisking.
6. Continue adding the remaining coconut milk, a tablespoonful at a time, until dough forms.
7. Mix in the cashew cheese and pimientos. (If the dough is too wet to handle, mix in a little bit more flour until it is manageable).
8. Place the dough on a lightly floured surface and flatten the dough into ½-inch thickness.
9. Use a 2 ½inch round cutter to cut out biscuits' pieces from the dough.
10. Gather, re-roll the dough once and continue cutting out biscuits.
11. Arrange the biscuits on the prepared pan and brush the tops with the melted butter.
12. Bake for 12-14 minutes, or until the biscuits are golden brown.
13. Cool and serve.

Nutrition:

Calories 1009 | Fats 71. 8g | Carbs 74. 8g | Protein 24. 5g

Breakfast Naan Bread with Mango Saffron Jam

Preparation Time: 5-15 minutes | Cooking Time: 40 minutes | Servings: 4

Ingredients:

For the naan bread:

- ¾ cup almond flour
- 1 tsp salt + extra for sprinkling
- 1 tsp baking powder
- 1/3 cup olive oil
- 2 cups boiling water
- 2 tbsp plant butter for frying

For the mango saffron jam:

- 4 cups heaped chopped mangoes
- 1 cup pure maple syrup
- 1 lemon, juiced
- A pinch of saffron powder
- 1 tsp cardamom powder

Directions:

For the naan bread:

1. In a large bowl, mix the almond flour, salt, and baking powder. Mix in the olive oil and
2. boiling water until smooth, thick batter forms. Allow the dough to rise for 5 minutes.
3. Form 6 to 8 balls out of the dough, place each on a baking paper and use your hands to
4. flatten the dough.
5. Working in batches, melt the plant butter in a large skillet and fry the dough on both sides
6. until set and golden brown on each side, 4 minutes per bread. Transfer to a plate and set aside
7. for serving.

For the mango saffron jam

1. Add the mangoes, maple syrup, lemon juice, and 3 tbsp of water in a medium pot and cook over medium heat until boiling, 5 minutes.
2. Mix in the saffron and cardamom powders and cook further over low heat until the mangoes are softened.
3. Mash the mangoes with the back of the spoon until fairly smooth with little chunks of mangoes in the jam.
4. Turn the heat off and cool completely.
5. Spoon the jam into sterilized jars and serve with the naan bread.

Nutrition:

Calories 766 | Fats 42. 7g | Carbs 93. 8g | Protein 7. 3g

Cauliflower and Potato Hash Browns

Preparation Time: 5-15 minutes | Cooking Time: 35 minutes | Servings: 4

Ingredients:

- 3 tbsp flax seed powder + 9 tbsp water
- 2 large potatoes, peeled and shredded
- 1 big head cauliflower, rinsed and riced
- ½ white onion, grated
- 1 tsp salt
- 1 tbsp black pepper
- 4 tbsp plant butter, for frying

Directions:

1. In a medium bowl, mix the flaxseed powder and water. Allow thickening for 5 minutes for the flax egg.
2. Add the potatoes, cauliflower, onion, salt, and black pepper to the flax egg and mix until well combined.
3. Allow sitting for 5 minutes to thicken.

4. Working in batches, melt 1 tbsp of plant butter in a non-stick skillet and add 4 scoops of the hash brown mixture to the skillet.
5. Make sure to have 1 to 2-inch intervals between each scoop.
6. Use the spoon to flatten the batter and cook until compacted and golden brown on the bottom part, 2 minutes.
7. Flip the hashbrowns and cook further for 2 minutes or until the vegetables are cooked and golden brown.
8. Transfer to a paper towel-lined plate to drain grease.
9. Make the remaining hashbrowns using the remaining ingredients.
10. Serve warm.

Nutrition:

Calories 265 | Fats 11. 9g | Carbs 36. 7g | Protein 5. 3g

Raspberry Raisin Muffins with Orange Glaze

Preparation Time: 5-15 minutes | Cooking Time: 40 minutes | Servings: 4

Ingredients:

For the muffins:

- 2 tbsp flax seed powder + 6 tbsp water
- 2 cups whole-wheat flour
- 1½ tsp baking powder
- A pinch salt
- ½ cup plant butter, room temperature
- 1 cup pure date sugar
- ½ cup oat milk
- 2 tsp vanilla extract
- 1 lemon, zested
- 1 cup dried raspberries

For the orange glaze:

- 2 tbsp orange juice
- 1 cup pure date sugar

Directions:

1. Preheat the oven to 400 F and grease 6 muffin cups with cooking spray.
2. In a small bowl, mix the flax seed powder with water and allow thickening for 5 minutes to make the flax egg.
3. In a medium bowl, mix the flour, baking powder, and salt.
4. In another bowl, cream the plant butter, date sugar, and flax egg.
5. Mix in the oat milk, vanilla, and lemon zest.
6. Combine both mixtures, fold in raspberries, and fill muffin cups two-thirds way up with the batter.
7. Bake until a toothpick inserted comes out clean, 20-25 minutes.
8. In a medium bowl, whisk orange juice and date sugar until smooth.
9. Remove the muffins when ready and transfer them to a wire rack to cool.
10. Drizzle the glaze on top to serve.

Nutrition:

Calories 700 | Fats 25. 5g | Carbs 115. 1g | Protein 10. 5g

Berry Cream Compote Over Crepes

Preparation Time: 5-15 minutes | Cooking Time: 35 minutes | Servings: 4

Ingredients:

For the berry cream:

- 1 knob plant butter
- 2 tbsp pure date sugar
- 1 tsp vanilla extract
- ½ cup fresh blueberries
- ½ cup fresh raspberries
- ½ cup whipped coconut cream

For the crepes:

- 2 tbsp flax seed powder + 6 tbsp water
- 1 tsp vanilla extract
- 1 tsp pure date sugar
- ¼ tsp salt
- 2 cups almond flour
- 1 ½ cups almond milk
- 1 ½ cups water

- 3 tbsp plant butter for frying

Directions:

1. Melt butter in a pot over low heat and mix in the date sugar, and vanilla.
2. Cook until the sugar melts and then toss in berries.
3. Allow softening for 2 3 minutes.
4. Set aside to cool.
5. In a medium bowl, mix the flax seed powder with water and allow thickening for 5 minutes to make the flax egg.
6. Whisk in the vanilla, date sugar, and salt.
7. Pour in a quarter cup of almond flour and whisk, then a quarter cup of almond milk, and mix until no lumps remain.
8. Repeat the mixing process with the remaining almond flour and almond milk in the same quantities until exhausted.
9. Mix in 1 cup of water until the mixture is runny like that of pancakes and add the remaining water until the mixture is lighter.
10. Brush a large non-stick skillet with some butter and place over medium heat to melt.
11. Pour 1 tablespoon of the batter into the pan and swirl the skillet quickly and all around to coat the pan with the batter.

12. Cook until the batter is dry and golden brown beneath, about 30 seconds.

13. Use a spatula to carefully flip the crepe and cook the other side until golden brown too.

14. Fold the crepe onto a plate and set aside.

15. Repeat making more crepes with the remaining batter until exhausted.

16. Plate the crepes, top with the whipped coconut cream, and the berry compote.

17. Serve immediately.

Nutrition:

Calories 339 | Fats 24. 5g | Carbs 30g | Protein 2. 3g

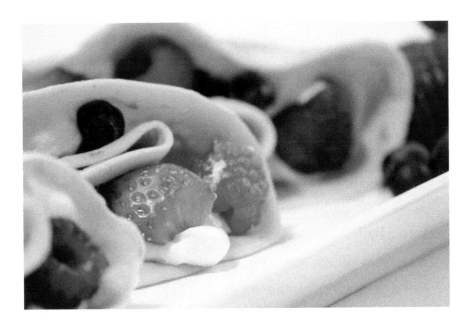

Irish Brown Bread

Preparation Time: 5-15 minutes | Cooking Time: 50 minutes | Servings: 4

Ingredients:

- 4 cups whole-wheat flour
- ¼ tsp salt
- ½ cup rolled oats
- 1 tsp baking soda
- 1 ¾ cups coconut milk, thick
- 2 tbsp pure maple syrup

Directions:

1. Preheat the oven to 400 F.
2. In a bowl, mix flour, salt, oats, and baking soda.
3. Add in coconut milk, maple syrup, and
4. whisk until dough forms.
5. Dust your hands with some flour and knead the dough into a ball.
6. Shape the dough into a circle and place on a baking sheet.
7. Cut a deep cross on the dough and bake in the oven for 15 minutes at 450 F.

8. Then, reduce the temperature to 400 F and bake further for 20 to 25 minutes or until a hollow sound is made when the bottom of the bread is tapped.
9. Slice and serve.

Nutrition:

Calories 963 | Fats 44. 4g | Carbs 125. 1g | Protein 22. 1g

Apple Cinnamon Muffins

Preparation Time: 5-15 minutes | Cooking Time: 40 minutes | Servings: 4

Ingredients:

For the muffins:

- 1 flax seed powder + 3 tbsp water
- 1 ½ cups whole-wheat flour
- ¾ cup pure date sugar
- 2 tsp baking powder
- ¼ tsp salt
- 1 tsp cinnamon powder
- 1/3 cup melted plant butter
- 1/3 cup flax milk
- 2 apples, peeled, cored, and chopped

For topping:

- 1/3 cup whole-wheat flour
- ½ cup pure date sugar
- ½ cup cold plant butter, cubed
- 1 ½ tsp cinnamon powder

Directions:

1. Preheat the oven to 400 F and grease 6 muffin cups with cooking spray.
2. In a bowl, mix the flax seed powder with water and allow thickening for 5 minutes to make the flax egg.
3. In a medium bowl, mix the flour, date sugar, baking powder, salt, and cinnamon powder.
4. Whisk in the butter, flax egg, flax milk, and then fold in the apples.
5. Fill the muffin cups twothirds way up with the batter.
6. In a small bowl, mix the remaining flour, date sugar, cold butter, and cinnamon powder.
7. Sprinkle the mixture on the muffin batter.
8. Bake for 20-minutes.
9. Remove the muffins onto a wire rack, allow cooling, and serve warm.

Nutrition:

Calories 1133 | Fats 74. 9g | Carbs 104. 3g | Protein 18g

Mixed Berry Walnut Yogurt

Preparation Time: 5-15 minutes | Cooking Time: 10 minutes | Servings: 4

Ingredients:

- 4 cups almond milk Dairy-Free yogurt, cold
- 2 tbsp pure malt syrup
- 2 cups mixed berries, halved or chopped
- ¼ cup chopped toasted walnuts

Directions:

1. In a medium bowl, mix the yogurt and malt syrup until well-combined.
2. Divide the mixture into 4 breakfast bowls.
3. Top with the berries and walnuts.
4. Enjoy immediately.

Nutrition:

Calories 326 | Fats 14. 3g | Carbs 38. 3g | Protein 12. 5g

Orange Butter Crepes

Preparation Time: 5-15 minutes | Cooking Time: 30 minutes | Servings: 4

Ingredients:

- 2 tbsp flax seed powder + 6 tbsp water
- 1 tsp vanilla extract
- 1 tsp pure date sugar
- ¼ tsp salt
- 2 cups almond flour
- 1½ cups oat milk
- ½ cup melted plant butter
- 3 tbsp fresh orange juice
- 3 tbsp plant butter for frying

Directions:

1. In a medium bowl, mix the flax seed powder with 1 cup water and allow thickening for 5 minutes to make the flax egg. Whisk in the vanilla, date sugar, and salt.
2. Pour in a quarter cup of almond flour and whisk, then a quarter cup of oat milk, and mix until no lumps remain.

3. Repeat the mixing process with the remaining almond flour and almond milk in the same quantities until exhausted.

4. Mix in the plant butter, orange juice, and half of the water until the mixture is runny like that of pancakes.

5. Add the remaining water until the mixture is lighter.

6. Brush a large non-stick skillet with some butter and place over medium heat to melt.

7. Pour 1 tablespoon of the batter into the pan and swirl the skillet quickly and all around to coat the pan with the batter.

8. Cook until the batter is dry and golden brown beneath, about 30 seconds.

9. Use a spatula to carefully flip the crepe and cook the other side until golden brown too.

10. Fold the crepe onto a plate and set aside.

11. Repeat making more crepes with the remaining batter until exhausted.

12. Drizzle some maple syrup on the crepes and serve.

Nutrition:

Calories 379 | Fats 35. 6g | Carbs 14. 8g | Protein 5. 6g

Creole Tofu Scramble

Preparation Time: 5-15 minutes | Cooking Time: 20 minutes | Servings: 4

Ingredients:

- 2 tbsp plant butter, for frying
- 1 (14 oz) pack firm tofu, pressed and crumbled
- 1 medium red bell pepper, deseeded and chopped
- 1 medium green bell pepper, deseeded and chopped
- 1 tomato, finely chopped
- 2 tbsp chopped fresh green onions
- Salt and black pepper to taste
- 1 tsp turmeric powder
- 1 tsp Creole seasoning
- ½ cup chopped baby kale
- ¼ cup grated plant-based Parmesan cheese

Directions:

1. Melt the plant butter in a large skillet over medium heat and add the tofu.

2. Cook with occasional stirring until the tofu is light golden brown while making sure not to break the tofu into tiny bits but to have scrambled egg resemblance, 5 minutes.

3. Stir in the bell peppers, tomato, green onions, salt, black pepper, turmeric powder, and Creole seasoning.

4. Sauté until the vegetables soften, 5 minutes.

5. Mix in the kale to wilt, 3 minutes and then, half of the plant-based Parmesan cheese.

6. Allow melting for 1 to 2 minutes and then turn the heat off.

7. Dish the food, top with the remaining cheese, and serve warm.

Nutrition:

Calories 258 | Fats 15. 9g | Carbs 12. 8g | Protein 20. 7g

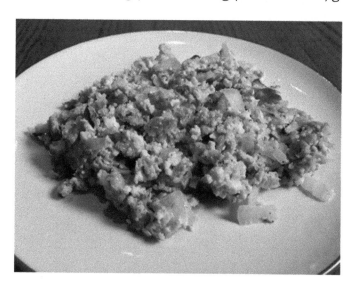

Mushroom Avocado Panini

Preparation Time: 5-15 minutes | Cooking Time: 30 minutes | Servings: 4

Ingredients:

- 1 tbsp olive oil
- 1 cup sliced white button mushrooms
- Salt and black pepper to taste
- 1 ripe avocado, pitted, peeled, and sliced
- 2 tbsp freshly squeezed lemon juice
- 1 tbsp chopped parsley
- ½ tsp pure maple syrup
- 8 slices whole-wheat ciabatta
- 4 oz sliced plant-based Parmesan cheese
- 1 tbsp olive oil

Directions:

1. Heat the olive oil in a medium skillet over medium heat and sauté the mushrooms until softened, 5 minutes.
2. Season with salt and black pepper.
3. Turn the heat off.
4. Preheat a panini press to medium heat, 3 to 5 minutes.

5. Mash the avocado in a medium bowl and mix in the lemon juice, parsley, and maple syrup.
6. Spread the mixture on 4 bread slices, divide the mushrooms and plant-based Parmesan cheese on top.
7. Cover with the other bread slices and brush the top with olive oil.
8. Grill the sandwiches one after another in the heated press until golden brown and the cheese melted.
9. Serve warm.

Nutrition:

Calories 338 | Fats 22. 4g | Carbs 25. 5g | Protein 12. 4g

Avocado Toast with Herbs and Peas

Preparation Time: 10 minutes | Cooking Time: 0 minute | Servings: 4

Ingredients:

- ½ of a medium avocado, peeled, pitted, mashed
- 6 slices of radish
- 2 tablespoons baby peas
- ¼ teaspoon ground black pepper
- 1 teaspoon chopped basil
- ¼ teaspoon salt
- 1/2 lemon, juiced
- 1 slice of bread, whole-grain, toasted

Directions:

1. Spread mashed avocado on one side of the toast and then top with peas, pressing them into the avocado.
2. Layer the toast with radish slices, season with salt and black pepper, sprinkle with basil and drizzle with lemon juice.

3. Serve straight away.

Nutrition:

Calories: 250 Cal |Fat: 12 g | Carbs: 22 g | Protein: 7 g | Fiber: 9 g

Small Sweet Potato Pancakes

Preparation Time: 20 minutes | Cooking Time: 0 minutes | Servings: 2

Ingredients:

- 1 clove of garlic
- 3 tablespoon wholemeal rice flour
- 1 pinch of nutmeg
- 3 tablespoons of water
- 150 g sweet potato
- 1 pinch of chili flakes
- 1 teaspoon oil
- Salt

Directions:

1. Peel the garlic clove and mash it with a fork.
2. Peel the sweet potato and grate it into small sticks with a grater.
3. Knead the sweet potato and garlic in a bowl with the rice flour and water, then season with chili flakes, salt, and nutmeg.
4. Heat the oil in a pan and form small buffers.

5. Fry these in the pan on both sides until golden brown.

6. Goes perfectly with tzatziki and other fresh dips.

Nutrition:

Calories: 209 |Fat: 15.4g |Carbs: 10.5g |Protein: 8.1g |Fiber: 3.2g

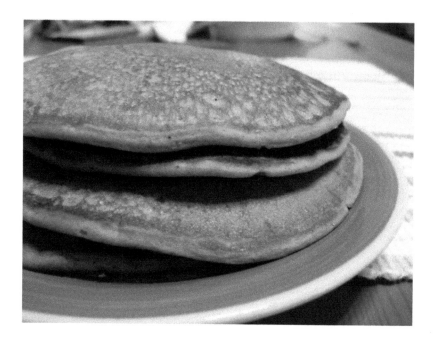

Tomato and Pesto Toast

Preparation Time: 5 minutes | Cooking Time: 0 minute | Servings: 4

Ingredients:

- 1 small tomato, sliced
- ¼ teaspoon ground black pepper
- 1 tablespoon vegan pesto
- 2 tablespoons hummus
- 1 slice of whole-grain bread, toasted
- Hemp seeds as needed for garnishing

Directions:

1. Spread hummus on one side of the toast, top with tomato slices and then drizzle with pesto.
2. Sprinkle black pepper on the toast along with hemp seeds and then serve straight away.

Nutrition:

- Calories: 214 Cal | Fat: 7.2 g |Carbs: 32 g | Protein: 6.5 g |Fiber: 3 g

Avocado and Sprout Toast

Preparation Time: 5 minutes | Cooking Time: 0 minute | Servings: 4

Ingredients:

- 1/2 of a medium avocado, sliced
- 1 slice of whole-grain bread, toasted
- 2 tablespoons sprouts
- 2 tablespoons hummus
- ¼ teaspoon lemon zest
- ½ teaspoon hemp seeds
- ¼ teaspoon red pepper flakes

Directions:

1. Spread hummus on one side of the toast and then top with avocado slices and sprouts.
2. Sprinkle with lemon zest, hemp seeds, and red pepper flakes, and then serve straight away.

Nutrition:

- Calories: 200 Cal | Fat: 10.5 g | Carbs: 22 g |Protein: 7 g |Fiber: 7 g

Apple and Honey Toast

Preparation Time: 5 minutes | Cooking Time: 0 minute | Servings: 4

Ingredients:

- ½ of a small apple, cored, sliced
- 1 slice of whole-grain bread, toasted
- 1 tablespoon honey
- 2 tablespoons hummus
- 1/8 teaspoon cinnamon

Directions:

1. Spread hummus on one side of the toast, top with apple slices and then drizzle with honey.
2. Sprinkle cinnamon on it and then serve straight away.

Nutrition:

Calories: 212 Cal | Fat: 7 g | Carbs: 35 g | Protein: 4 g | Fiber: 5.5 g

Zucchini Pancakes

Preparation Time: 10 minutes | Cooking Time: 15 minutes | Servings: 4

Ingredients:

- 2 cups zucchini
- 1/4 cup onion
- 1 tablespoon all-purpose white flour
- 1 teaspoon herb seasoning
- 1 egg 1 tablespoon olive oil
- 1/8 teaspoon salt

Directions:

1. Grate onion and zucchini into a bowl and stir to combine.
2. Place the zucchini mixture on a clean kitchen towel.
3. Twist and squeeze out as much liquid as possible.
4. Return to the bowl.
5. Mix flour, salt, and herb seasoning in a small bowl.
6. Add egg and mix; stir into zucchini and
7. onion mixture.
8. Form 4 patties.
9. Heat oil over high heat in a large non-stick frying pan.

10. Lower heat to medium and place zucchini patties into the pan.

11. Sauté until brown, turning once.

Nutrition:

Calories 65, | Total Fat 4.7g | Saturated Fat 0.9g | Cholesterol 41mg | Sodium 97mg | Total Carbohydrate 4.1g | Dietary Fiber 0.8g| Total Sugars 1.4g | Protein 2.3g | Calcium 16mg | Iron 1mg | Potassium 175mg | Phosphorus 24mg

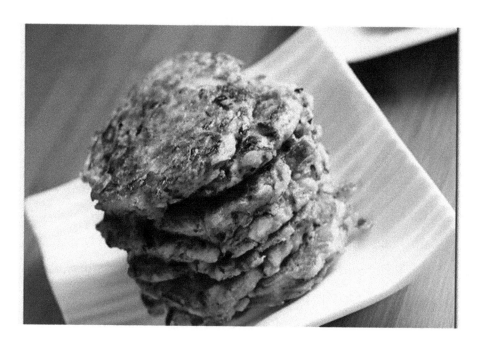

Savory Spinach and Mushroom Crepes

Preparation Time: 60 minutes | Cooking Time: 30-120 minutes | Servings: 4

Ingredients:

For the crepes:

- 1 ¾ cup rolled oats
- 1 tsp pink Himalayan salt
- 1 ½ cup of soy milk
- 2 tbsp olive oil
- 1 tbsp almond butter
- ½ tsp nutmeg
- 2 tbsp egg replacement

For the filling:

- 1 lb button mushrooms
- 10 oz fresh spinach, finely chopped
- 4 oz crumbled tofu
- 1 tbsp chia seeds
- 1 tbsp fresh rosemary, finely chopped
- 1 garlic clove, crushed

- 2 tbsp olive oil

Directions:

1. First, prepare the crepes.
2. Combine all dry ingredients in a large bowl.
3. Add milk, butter, nutmeg, olive oil, and egg replacement.
4. Mix well with a hand mixer on high speed.
5. Transfer to a food processor and process until completely smooth.
6. Grease a large non-stick pancake pan with some oil.
7. Pour 1 cup of the mixture into the pan and cook for one minute on each side.
8. Plug your Pressure pot and press the _Sauté' button.
9. Grease the stainless steel insert with some oil and add mushrooms.
10. Cook for 5 minutes, stirring constantly.
11. Now add spinach, tofu, rosemary, and garlic.
12. Continue to cook for another 5 minutes.
13. Remove the mixture from the pot and stir in chia seeds.
14. Let it sit for 10 minutes.
15. Meanwhile, grease a small baking pan with some oil and line with parchment paper.
16. Divide the mushroom mixture between crepes and roll-up. Gently transfer to a prepared baking pan.
17. Wrap the pan with aluminum foil and set aside.

18. Pour 1 cup of water into your Pressure pot and set the steam rack. Put the pan on top and seal the lid.
19. Press the _Manual' button and set the timer for 10 minutes.
20. When done, release the pressure naturally, and open the lid.
21. Optionally, sprinkle with some dried oregano before serving.

Nutrition:

Calories:680 | Total Fat:71.8g | Saturated Fat:20.9g | Total Carbs:10g | Dietary Fiber:7g | Sugar:2g | Protein:3g | Sodium:525mg

Spinach Pesto Pasta

Preparation Time: 05 minutes | Cooking Time: 10 minutes | Servings: 2

Ingredients:

- 1cup pasta
- 2 cups spinach, chopped
- ¼ cup of coconut oil
- ½ large lemon
- ¼ teaspoon garlic powder
- 1/8 cup chopped pecans
- ¼ cup goat cheese, grated
- ¼ teaspoon salt
- Freshly cracked pepper to taste
- 2 oz. mozzarella (optional)

Directions:

1. Add the chopped and washed spinach to a food processor along with the coconut oil, 1/4 cup juice from the lemon, garlic powder, pecans, goat cheese, salt, and pepper.
2. Purée the mixture until smooth and bright green.
3. Add more oil if needed to allow the mixture to become a thick, smooth sauce.

4. Taste the pesto and adjust the salt, pepper, or lemon juice to your liking. Set the pesto aside.
5. Add pasta, water, and pesto, coconut oil into Pressure pot.
6. Place lid on Pressure pot and lock into place to seal.
7. Pressure Cook on High Pressure for 4 minutes.
8. Use Quick Pressure Release.
9. Add mozzarella cheese and serve.

Nutrition:

Calories 534 | Total Fat 35. 8g | Saturated Fat 27. 7g | Cholesterol 65mg | Sodium 514mg | Total Carbohydrate 39g | Dietary Fiber 1. 2g | Total Sugars 0. 7g | Protein 17. 5g

Paprika Pumpkin Pasta

Preparation Time: 05 minutes | Cooking Time: 10 minutes | Servings: 2

Ingredients:

- ¼ cup of coconut oil
- ½ onion
- ½ tablespoon butter
- ½ teaspoon garlic
- ¼ teaspoon paprika
- 1 cup pumpkin purée
- 5 cups vegetable broth
- ¼ teaspoon salt
- Freshly cracked pepper
- 1 cup pasta
- 1/8 cup coconut cream
- 1/4 cup grated mozzarella cheese

Directions:

1. Add the coconut oil to the Pressure pot, hit —Sauté‖, Add butter and onion until it is soft and transparent.

2. Add the garlic and paprika to the onion and sauté for about one minute more. Finally, add the pumpkin purée, vegetable broth, salt, and pepper to the Pressure pot and stir until the ingredients are combined and smooth.
3. Add pasta, then place a lid on the Pressure pot and lock it into place to seal.
4. Pressure Cook on High Pressure for 4 minutes.
5. Use Quick Pressure Release.
6. Add coconut cream and mozzarella cheese.

Nutrition:

Calories 327 | Total Fat 8. 9g | Saturated Fat 4. 4g | Cholesterol 67mg | Sodium 931mg | Total Carbohydrate 49g | Dietary Fiber 4. 7g | Total Sugars 5. 7g | Protein 13. 5g

Creamy Mushroom Herb Pasta

Preparation Time: 05 minutes | Cooking Time: 10 minutes | Servings: 2

Ingredients:

- ¼ cup of coconut oil
- ½ cup mushrooms
- ½ teaspoon garlic powder
- 1 1/2 tablespoon butter
- 1 1/2 tablespoon coconut flour
- 1 cup vegetable broth
- 1 sprig fresh thyme
- ½ teaspoon basil
- Salt and pepper to taste

Directions:

1. Add the coconut oil to the Pressure pot, hit ─Sauté‖, add butter, when the butter melts add garlic powder, add the sliced mushrooms and continue to cook until the mushrooms have turned dark brown and all of the moisture they release has evaporated.

2. Add the flour, Whisk the vegetable broth into the Pressure pot with the flour and mushrooms.
3. Add the thyme, basil, and some freshly cracked pepper.
4. Then add pasta, place the lid on the pot and lock it into place to seal.
5. Pressure Cook on High Pressure for 4 minutes.
6. Use Quick Pressure Release.
7. Serve and enjoy.

Nutrition:

Calories 107 | Total Fat 7. 5g | Saturated Fat 4. 8g | Cholesterol 15mg | Sodium 439mg | Total Carbohydrate 5. 7g | Dietary Fiber 2. 8g | Total Sugars 1. 3g | Protein 4. 2g

Cabbage and Noodles

Preparation Time: 05 minutes | Cooking Time: 05 minutes | Servings: 2

Ingredients:

- 1 cup wide egg noodles
- 1 1/2 tablespoon butter
- 1small onion
- 1/2 head green cabbage, shredded
- Salt and pepper to taste

Directions:

1. Add egg noodles, butter, water, onion, green cabbage, pepper, and salt to Pressure pot.
2. Place lid on Pressure pot and lock into place to seal.
3. Pressure Cook on High Pressure for 4 minutes.
4. Use Quick Pressure Release.
5. Serve and enjoy.

Nutrition:

Calories183 | Total Fat 6. 8g | Saturated Fat 3. 9g | Cholesterol 31mg | Sodium 78mg | Total Carbohydrate 27. 2g | Dietary Fiber 5. 9g | Total Sugars 7. 6g| Protein 5. 4g

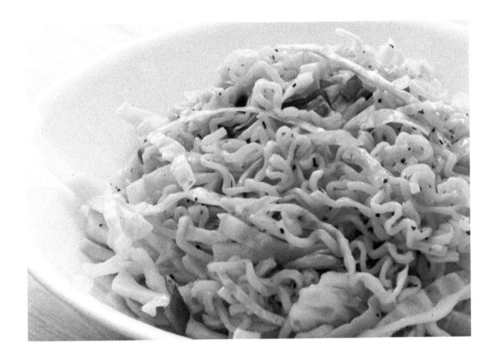

Lemon Garlic Broccoli Macaroni

Ingredients:

- 1 cup macaroni
- ½ cup broccoli
- 1 tablespoon butter
- ½ teaspoon garlic powder
- 1 lemon
- Salt and pepper to taste
- Enough water

Directions:

1. Add macaroni, butter, water, broccoli, lemon, garlic powder, and salt to Pressure pot.
2. Place the lid on the pot and lock it into place to seal.
3. Pressure Cook on High Pressure for 4 minutes.
4. Use Quick Pressure Release.

Nutrition:

Calories 254 | Total Fat 7. 4g | Saturated Fat 3. 9g | Cholesterol 62mg | Sodium 66mg | Total Carbohydrate 39. 8g | Dietary Fiber 1. 5g | Total Sugars 1. 3g | Protein 8. 4g

Basil Spaghetti Pasta

Preparation Time: 05 minutes | Cooking Time: 05 minutes | Servings: 2

Ingredients:

- ½ teaspoon garlic powder
- 1 cup spaghetti
- 2 large eggs
- ¼ cup grated Parmesan cheese
- Freshly cracked pepper
- Salt and pepper to taste
- Handful fresh basil
- Enough water

Directions:

1. In a medium bowl, whisk together the eggs, 1/2 cup of the Parmesan cheese, and a generous dose of freshly cracked pepper.
2. Add spaghetti, water, basil, garlic powder, pepper, and salt to Pressure pot.
3. Place lid on Pressure pot and lock into place to seal.
4. Pressure Cook on High Pressure for 4 minutes.

5. Use Quick Pressure Release.

6. Pour the eggs and Parmesan mixture over the hot pasta.

Nutrition:

Calories216 | Total Fat 2. 3g | Saturated Fat 0. 7g | Cholesterol 49mg | Sodium 160mg | Total Carbohydrate 36g | Dietary Fiber 0. 1g | Total Sugars 0. 4g | Protein 12. 2g

Parsley Hummus Pasta

Ingredients:

- ½ cup chickpeas
- 1/8 cup coconut oil
- ½ fresh lemon
- 1/8 cup tahini
- ½ teaspoon garlic powder
- 1/8 teaspoon cumin
- 1/4 teaspoon salt
- 1 green onion
- 1/8 bunch fresh parsley, or to taste
- 1 cup pasta
- Enough water

Directions:

1. Drain the chickpeas and add them to a food processor along with the coconut oil, juice from the lemon, tahini, garlic powder, cumin, and salt.
2. Pulse the ingredients, adding a small amount of water if needed to keep it moving, until the hummus is smooth.
3. Slice the green onion (both white and green ends) and pull the parsley leaves from the stems.

4. Add the green onion and parsley to the hummus in the food processor and process again until only small flecks of green remain.

5. Taste the hummus and adjust the salt, lemon, or garlic if needed.

6. Add pasta, water into Pressure pot.

7. Place the lid on the pot and lock it into place to seal.

8. Pressure Cook on High Pressure for 4 minutes.

9. Use Quick Pressure Release.

10. In Sauté mode add hummus to pasta.

11. When it mixes, turn off the switch of Pressure pot.

12. Serve and enjoy.

Nutrition:

• Calories 582 | Total Fat 26. 3g | Saturated Fat 13. 5g | Cholesterol 47mg | Sodium 338mg | Total Carbohydrate 71g | Dietary Fiber 10. 8g | Total Sugars 6. 1g | Protein 19. 9g

Creamy Spinach Artichoke Pasta

Preparation Time: 05 minutes | Cooking Time: 05 minutes | Servings: 2

Ingredients:

- 1 tablespoon butter
- ¼ teaspoon garlic powder
- 1 cup vegetable broth
- 1 cup of coconut milk
- ¼ teaspoon salt
- Freshly cracked pepper
- ½ cup pasta
- 1/4 cup fresh baby spinach
- ½ cup quartered artichoke hearts
- 1/8 cup grated Parmesan cheese

Directions:

1. In the Pressure pot, hit —Sauté‖, add butter when it melts, add garlic powder just until it's tender and fragrant.
2. Add the vegetable broth, coconut milk, salt, some freshly cracked pepper, and pasta.

3. Place the lid on the pot and lock it into place to seal.

4. Pressure Cook on High Pressure for 4 minutes.

5. Use Quick Pressure Release.

6. Add the spinach, a handful at a time, to the hot pasta and toss it in the pasta until it wilts into

7. Pressure pot in Sauté mode. Stir the chopped artichoke hearts into the pasta.

8. Sprinkle grated Parmesan over the pasta, then stir slightly to incorporate the Parmesan.

9. Top with an additional Parmesan then serve.

Nutrition:

Calories 457 | Total Fat 36. 2g | Saturated Fat 29. 6g | Cholesterol 40mg, Sodium 779mg | Total Carbohydrate 27. 6g | Dietary Fiber 4g | Total Sugars 4. 7g | Protein 10. 3g

Easy Spinach Ricotta Pasta

Preparation Time: 05 minutes | Cooking Time: 10 minutes | Servings: 2

Ingredients:

- ½ cup pasta
- 1 cup vegetable broth
- 1/2 lb. uncooked tagliatelle
- 1 tablespoon coconut oil
- ½ teaspoon garlic powder
- ¼ cup almond milk
- ½ cup whole milk ricotta
- 1/8 teaspoon salt
- Freshly cracked pepper
- ¼ cup chopped spinach

Directions:

1. Add the vegetable broth, tagliatelle, spinach, salt, some freshly cracked pepper, and the pasta.
2. Place lid on Pressure pot and lock into place to seal.
3. Pressure Cook on High Pressure for 4 minutes.
4. Use Quick Pressure Release.

5. Prepare the ricotta sauce.

6. Mince the garlic and add it to a large skillet with coconut oil.

7. Cook over Medium-Low heat for 1-2 minutes, or just until soft and fragrant (but not browned).

8. Add the almond milk and ricotta, then stir until relatively smooth (the ricotta may be slightly grainy).

9. Allow the sauce to heat through and come to a low simmer.

10. The sauce will thicken slightly as it simmers.

11. Once it's thick enough to coat the spoon (3-5 minutes), season with salt and pepper.

12. Add the cooked and drained pasta to the sauce and toss to coat.

13. If the sauce becomes too thick or dry, add a small amount of the reserved pasta cooking water.

14. Serve warm.

Nutrition:

Calories277 | Total Fat 18. 9g | Saturated Fat 15. 2g | Cholesterol 16mg |, Sodium 191mg, Total

Roasted Red Pepper Pasta

Preparation Time: 05 minutes | Cooking Time: 05 minutes | Servings: 2

Ingredients:

- 2 cups vegetable broth
- ½ cup spaghetti
- 1 small onion
- ½ teaspoon garlic minced
- ½ cup roasted red peppers
- ½ cup roasted diced tomatoes
- ¼ tablespoon dried mint
- 1/8 teaspoon crushed red pepper
- Freshly cracked black pepper
- ½ cup goat cheese

Directions:

1. In an Pressure pot, combine the vegetable broth, onion, garlic, red pepper slices, diced tomatoes, mint, crushed red pepper, and some freshly cracked black pepper.
2. Stir these ingredients to combine.
3. Add spaghetti to the Pressure pot.

4. Place lid on Pressure pot and lock into place to seal.

5. Pressure Cook on High Pressure for 4 minutes.

6. Use Quick Pressure Release.

7. Divide the goat cheese into tablespoon-sized pieces, then add them to the Pressure pot.

8. Stir the pasta until the cheese melts in and creates a smooth sauce.

9. Serve hot.

Nutrition:

Calories198 | Total Fat 4. 9g | Saturated Fat 2. 2g | Cholesterol 31mg | Sodium 909mg | Total Carbohydrate 26. 8g | Dietary Fiber 1. 9g | Total Sugars 5. 6g | Protein 11. 9g

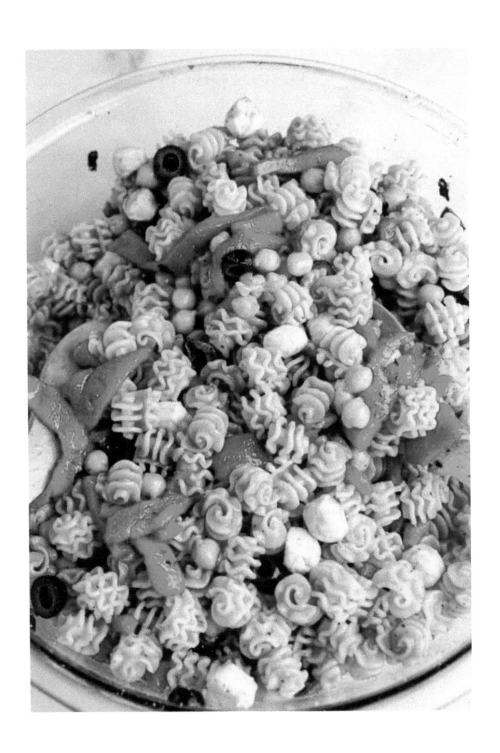

Cheese Beetroot Greens Macaroni

Preparation Time: 05 minutes | Cooking Time: 05 minutes | Servings: 2

Ingredients:

- 1 tablespoon butter
- 1 clove garlic minced
- 1 cup button mushrooms
- ½ bunch beetroot greens
- ½ cup vegetable broth
- ½ cup macaroni
- ¼ teaspoon salt
- ½ cup grated Parmesan cheese
- Freshly cracked pepper

Directions:

1. In the Pressure pot, hit —Sauté‖, add butter, garlic and slice the mushrooms.
2. Add the beetroot greens to the pot along with 1/2 cup vegetable broth.

3. Stir the beetroot greens as it cooks until it is fully wilted.

4. Add vegetable broth, macaroni, salt, and pepper.

5. Place lid on Pressure pot and lock into place to seal.

6. Pressure Cook on High Pressure for 4 minutes.

7. Use Quick Pressure Release.

8. Add grated Parmesan cheese.

Nutrition:

Calories 147 | Total Fat 8g | Saturated Fat 4. 8g | Cholesterol 23mg | Sodium 590mg | Total Carbohydrate 12. 7g | Dietary Fiber 1g | Total Sugars 1. 5g | Protein 6. 5g

Pastalaya

Preparation Time: 05 minutes | Cooking Time: 05 minutes | Servings: 2

Ingredients:

- ½ tablespoon avocado oil
- ½ teaspoon garlic powder
- 1 diced tomato
- ¼ teaspoon dried basil
- ¼ teaspoon smoked paprika
- ¼ teaspoon dried rosemary
- Freshly cracked pepper
- 1 cup vegetable broth
- ½ cup of water
- 1 cup orzo pasta
- 1 tablespoon coconut cream
- ½ bunch fresh coriander

Directions:

1. In the Pressure pot, place the garlic powder and avocado oil, sauté for 15 seconds, or until the garlic is fragrant.

2. Add diced tomatoes, basil, smoked paprika, rosemary, freshly cracked pepper, and orzo pasta to the Pressure pot.
3. Finally, add the vegetable broth and ½ cup of water, and stir until everything is evenly combined.
4. Place the lid on the Pressure pot, and bring the toggle switch into the −Sealing‖ position.
5. Press Manual or Pressure Cook and adjust the time for 5 minutes.
6. When the five minutes are up, do a Natural-release for 5 minutes and then move the toggle switch to −Venting‖ to release the rest of the pressure in the pot.
7. Remove the lid.
8. If the mixturelooks watery, press −Sauté‖ and bring the mixture up to a boil and let it boil for a few minutes. It will thicken as it boils.
9. Add the coconut cream and leek to the Pressure pot, stir and let warm through for a few minutes.
10. Serve and garnish with coriander toast. Enjoy!

Nutrition:

Calories 351 | Total Fat 6. 8g | Saturated Fat 3. 5g | Cholesterol 56mg | Sodium 869mg

Pasta with Peppers

Preparation Time: 5 minutes | Cooking Time: 15 minutes | Servings: 2

Ingredients:

- 1 1/2 cups spaghetti sauce
- 1 cup vegetable broth
- ½ tablespoon dried Italian seasoning blend
- 1 cup bell pepper strips
- 1 cup dried pasta
- 1 cup shredded Romano cheese

Directions:

1. Press the button Sauté.
2. Set it for High, and set the time for 10 minutes.
3. Mix the sauce, broth, and seasoning blend in a Pressure pot. Cook, turn off the Sauté
4. function; stir in the bell pepper strips and pasta.
5. Lock the lid onto the pot.
6. Press Pressure Cook on Max Pressure for 5 minutes with the Keep Warm setting off.

7. Use the Quick Release method to bring the pot pressure back to normal.

8. Unlatch the lid and open the cooker.

9. Stir in the shredded Romano cheese.

10. Set the lid askew over the pot and set aside for 5 minutes to melt the cheese and let the pasta continue to absorb excess liquid.

11. Serve by the big spoon.

Nutrition:

Calories 291 | Total Fat 6. 2g | Saturated Fat 2. 9g | Cholesterol 61mg | Sodium 994mg | Total Carbohydrate 43. 7g | Dietary Fiber 1g | Total Sugars 3. 5g | Protein 15. 1g

Fresh Tomato Mint Pasta

Preparation Time: 05 minutes | Cooking Time: 10 minutes | Servings: 2

Ingredients:

- 1 cup pasta
- 1 tablespoon coconut oil
- ½ teaspoon garlic powder
- 1 tomato
- ½ tablespoon butter
- ¼ cup fresh mint
- ¼ cup of coconut milk
- Salt & pepper to taste
- Enough water

Directions:

1. Add the coconut oil to the Pressure pot hit —Sauté‖, add in the garlic, and stir.
2. Add the tomatoes and a pinch of salt.
3. Then add mint and pepper.
4. Next, add coconut milk, butter, and water.
5. Stir well, lastly, add in the pasta.

6. Secure the lid and hit —Keep Warm/Cancel‖ and then hit —Manual‖ or —Pressure Cook‖ High Pressure for 6 minutes.

7. Quick-release when done.

8. Enjoy.

Nutrition:

Calories 350 | Total Fat 18. 5g | Saturated Fat 14. 3g | Cholesterol 54mg | Sodium 47mg | Total Carbohydrate 39. 4g | Dietary Fiber 1. 9g | Total Sugars 2g | Protein 8. 7g

Corn and Chiles Fusilli

Preparation Time: 05 minutes | Cooking Time: 05 minutes | Servings: 2

Ingredients:

- ½ tablespoon butter
- 1 tablespoon garlic minced
- Salt and pepper to taste
- 2 oz. can green chills
- ½ cup frozen corn kernels
- ¼ teaspoon cumin
- 1/8 teaspoon paprika
- 1 cup fusilli
- 1 cup vegetable broth
- ¼ cup coconut cream
- 2 leeks, sliced
- 1/8 bunch parsley
- 1 oz. shredded mozzarella cheese

Directions:

1. In the Pressure pot, add butter when butter melt, place the minced garlic, salt, and pepper, then press Sauté on the Pressure pot.

2. Add the can of green chills (with juices), frozen corn kernels, cumin, and paprika.

3. Add the uncooked fusilli and vegetable broth to the Pressure pot.

4. Place the lid on the Pressure pot, and bring the toggle switch into the −Sealing‖ position.

5. Press Manual or Pressure Cook and adjust the time for 5 minutes.

6. When the five minutes are up, do a Natural-release for 5 minutes and then move the toggle switch to −Venting‖ to release the rest of the pressure in the pot.

7. Remove the lid.

8. If the mixture looks watery, press −Sauté‖, and bring the mixture up to a boil and let it boil for a few minutes.

9. Then add the coconut cream and stir until it has fully coated the pasta.

10. Stir in most of the sliced leek and parsley, reserving a little to sprinkle over top, mozzarella on top of the pasta.

Nutrition:

Calories 399 | Total Fat 14. 4g | Saturated Fat 10g | Cholesterol 15mg | Sodium 531mg | Total Carbohydrate 56. 2g | Dietary Fiber 4. 9g |Total Sugars 7. 2g | Protein 15. 4g

Creamy Penne with Vegetables

- Preparation Time: 05 minutes | Cooking Time: 10 minutes | Servings: 2

Ingredients:

- ½ tablespoon butter
- 1 cup penne
- 1 small onion
- ½ teaspoon garlic powder
- 1 carrot
- ½ red bell pepper
- ½ pumpkin
- 2 cups vegetable broth
- 2 oz. coconut cream
- 1/8 cup grated Parmesan cheese
- 1/8 teaspoon salt and pepper to taste
- Dash hot sauce, optional
- ¼ cup cauliflower florets

Directions:

1. Set Pressure pot to Sauté.
2. Add the butter and allow it to melt.

3. Add the onion and garlic powder and cook for 2 minutes.
4. Stir regularly.
5. Add the carrot, red pepper and pumpkin, and cauliflower to the pot.
6. Add penne, vegetable broth, coconut cream, salt, and pepper then add hot sauce.
7. Lock the lid and make sure the vent is closed.
8. Set Pressure pot to Manual or Pressure Cook on High Pressure for 10 minutes.
9. When cooking time ends, release pressure and wait for steam to completely stop before opening the lid.
10. Stir in cheese, sprinkle a bit on top of the pasta when you serve it.

Nutrition:

Calories 381 | Total Fat 13. 2g | Saturated Fat 8. 7g | Cholesterol 56mg | Sodium 1006mg | Total Carbohydrate 52. 3g | Dietary Fiber 4. 7g | Total Sugars 8. 6g | Protein 15. 3g

Pasta with Eggplant Sauce

Preparation Time: 05 minutes | Cooking Time: 10 minutes | Servings: 2

Ingredients:

- 1 tablespoon coconut oil
- 2 cloves garlic
- 1 small onion
- 1 medium eggplant
- 1 cup diced tomatoes
- 1 tablespoon tomato sauce
- ¼ teaspoon dried thyme
- ½ teaspoon honey
- Pinch paprika
- Freshly cracked pepper
- ¼ salt and pepper, or to taste
- 6 oz. spaghetti
- 2 cups vegetable broth
- Handful fresh coriander, chopped

Directions:

1. Set Pressure pot to Sauté.

2. Add the coconut oil and allow it to melt.

3. Add the onion and garlic and cook for 2 minutes or until the onion is soft and transparent.

4. Add eggplant, diced tomatoes, tomato sauce, thyme, honey, paprika, and freshly cracked pepper.

5. Stir them well to combine.

6. Add spaghetti, and vegetable broth, salt, and pepper.

7. Lock the lid and make sure the vent is closed.

8. Set Pressure pot to Manual or Pressure Cook on High Pressure for 10 minutes.

9. When cooking time ends, release pressure and wait for steam to completely stop before opening the lid.

10. Top each serving with grated goat and a sprinkle of fresh coriander.

Nutrition:

Calories 306 | Total Fat 18g | Saturated Fat 12. 9g | Cholesterol 30mg | Sodium 188mg | Total Carbohydrate 27g | Dietary Fiber 12. 6g 45% | Total Sugars 13. 9g | Protein 14. 2g

Creamy Pesto Pasta with Tofu & Broccoli

Preparation Time: 05 minutes | Cooking Time: 10 minutes | Servings: 2

Ingredients:

- 4 oz. Farfalle pasta
- 4 oz. frozen broccoli florets
- ½ tablespoon coconut oil
- ½ cup tofu
- ¼ cup basil pesto
- ¼ cup vegetable broth
- 2 oz. heavy cream

Directions:

1. In the Pressure pot, add Farfalline pasta, broccoli, coconut oil, tofu, basil pesto, vegetable broth.
2. Cover the Pressure pot and lock it in.
3. Set the Manual or Pressure Cook timer for 10 minutes.
4. Make sure the timer is set to ―Sealing‖.

5. Once the timer reaches zero, quickly release the pressure. Add heavy cream.

6. Enjoy.

Nutrition:

Calories 383 | Total Fat 17. 8g | Saturated Fat 10. 1g | Cholesterol 39mg | Sodium 129mg | Total Carbohydrate 44g | Dietary Fiber 2. 4g | Total Sugars 3. 2g | Protein 13. 6g

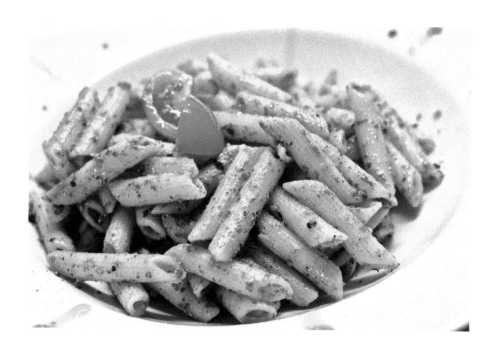

Chili Cheese Cottage Cheese Mac

Preparation Time: 05 minutes | Cooking Time: 12 minutes | Servings: 2

Ingredients:

- ½ tablespoon butter
- 1 cup cottage cheese
- ½ teaspoon garlic powder
- 1 small onion
- 1 tablespoon coconut flour
- ½ tablespoon chili powder
- ¼ teaspoon smoked paprika
- ¼ teaspoon dried basil
- 1 cup tomato paste
- 2 cups vegetable broth
- 1 cup dry macaroni
- ½ cup shredded sharp cheddar

Directions:

1. Set the Pressure pot to Sauté.
2. Add butter and wait one minute to heat up.
3. Add the cottage cheese, sauté for one minute.

4. Stir often.

5. Add coconut flour, onion, and garlic powder.

6. Add the chili powder, smoked paprika, basil, tomato paste, and 2 cups of vegetable broth.

7. Add the dry macaroni and cottage cheese.

8. Stir well.

9. Cover the Pressure pot and lock it in.

10. Set the Manual or Pressure Cook timer for 10 minutes.

11. Make sure the timer is set to—Sealing‖.

12. Once the timer reaches zero, quickly release the pressure.

13. Add shredded sharp cheddar cheese and enjoy.

Nutrition:

Calories 509 | Total Fat 11. 3g | Saturated Fat 6. 4g | Cholesterol 23mg | Sodium 1454mg | Total Carbohydrate 70. 3g | Dietary Fiber 10. 8g | Total Sugars 20. 5g | Protein 34. 8g

Spicy Cauliflower Pasta

Preparation Time: 05 minutes | Cooking Time: 10 minutes | Servings: 2

Ingredients:

- 1 tablespoon coconut oil
- 1 teaspoon garlic powder
- ¼ teaspoon paprika
- ½ cup cauliflower florets
- ½ cup broccoli florets
- 1 cup bow tie pasta
- Salt & pepper to taste
- 1 cup vegetable broth

Directions:

1. In the Pressure pot, set the Sauté button and add coconut oil when oil is hot, place garlic powder, paprika, cauliflower florets, broccoli florets, salt, and pepper.
2. Sauté the mixture untilit's cooked thoroughly.
3. Add the vegetable broth, and dry bow tie pasta.
4. Mix very well and place the lid on the Pressure pot, and bring the toggle switch into the ─Sealing‖ position.

5. Press Manual or Pressure Cook and adjust the time for 5 minutes.
6. When the five minutes are up, do a Natural-release for 5 minutes and then move the toggle switch to —Venting‖ to release the rest of the pressure in the pot.
7. Remove the lid. If the mixture looks watery, press —Sauté‖, and bring the mixture up to a boil and let it boil for a few minutes. It will thicken as it boils.
8. Serve and enjoy!

Nutrition:

Calories298 | Total Fat 10. 4g | Saturated Fat 7. 2g | Cholesterol 50mg | Sodium 426mg | Total Carbohydrate 39. 6g | Dietary Fiber 1. 5g | Total Sugars 1. 8g |Protein 12. 2g

Tasty Mac and Cheese

Preparation Time: 05 minutes | Cooking Time: 10 minutes | Servings: 2

Ingredients:

- ½ cup of soy milk
- 1 cup dry macaroni
- Enough water
- ½ cup shredded mozzarella cheese
- ¼ teaspoon salt
- ¼ teaspoon Dijon mustard
- 1/8 teaspoon red chili powder

Directions:

1. Add macaroni, soy milk, water, and salt, chili powder, Dijon mustard to the Pressure pot.
2. Place lid on Pressure pot and lock into place to seal.
3. Pressure Cook on High Pressure for 4 minutes.
4. Use Quick Pressure Release.
5. Stir cheese into macaroni and then stir in the cheeses until melted and combined.

Nutrition:

Calories 210 | Total Fat 3g, Saturated Fat 1g | Cholesterol 4mg | Sodium 374mg | Total Carbohydrate 35. 7g | Dietary Fiber 1. 8g | Total Sugars 3. 6g | Protein 9. 6g

Jackfruit and Red Pepper Pasta

- Preparation Time: 05 minutes | Cooking Time: 17 minutes | Servings: 2

Ingredients:

- ½ cup gnocchi
- 1/8 cup avocado oil
- ½ tablespoon garlic powder
- 1/2 teaspoon crushed red pepper
- ½ bunch fresh mint
- ½ cup jackfruit
- Salt to taste
- Enough water

Directions:

1. Set Pressure pot to Sauté.
2. Add the avocado oil and allow it to sizzle.
3. Add the garlic powder and cook for 2 minutes.
4. Stir regularly.
5. Add jackfruit and cook until about 4 - 5 minutes.
6. Add gnocchi, water, fresh mint, salt, and red pepper into Pressure pot.

7. Lock the lid and make sure the vent is closed.

8. Set Pressure pot to Manual or Pressure Cook on High PRESSURE for 10 minutes.

9. When cooking time ends, release pressure and wait for steam to completely stop before opening the lid.

10. Enjoy.

Nutrition:

Calories 110 | Total Fat 2. 3g | Saturated Fat 0. 4g | Cholesterol 0mg | Sodium 168mg | Total Carbohydrate 21. 5g | Dietary Fiber 2. 5g | Total Sugars 0. 6g | Protein 2. 3g

Creamy Mushroom Pasta with Broccoli

Preparation Time: 05 minutes | Cooking Time: 12 minutes | Servings: 2

Ingredients:

- 1 tablespoon coconut oil
- 1 small onion
- ½ teaspoon garlic powder
- 1 cup mushrooms
- 1 tablespoon coconut flour
- 1 cup of water
- ¼ cup red wine
- 1/8 cup coconut cream
- ¼ teaspoon dried basil
- Salt and pepper to taste
- 1/8 bunch fresh cilantro
- ½ cup mozzarella cheese
- 4 oz. pasta
- ½ cup broccoli

Directions:

1. Set Pressure pot to Sauté.
2. Add the coconut oil and allow it to sizzle.
3. Add coconut flour and mushrooms, sauté for 2 minutes.
4. Stir regularly.
5. It will coat the mushrooms and will begin to turn golden in color.
6. Just make sure to keep stirring so that the flour does not burn.
7. Combine water along with the red wine, basil, salt, and pepper.
8. Whisk until no flour lumps remain.
9. Add pasta, broccoli, cilantro, onion, and garlic powder.
10. Lock the lid and make sure the vent is closed.
11. Set Pressure pot to Manual or Pressure Cook on High Pressure for 10 minutes.
12. cooking time ends, release pressure and wait for steam to completely stop before opening the lid.
13. Stir in cheese and coconut cream.
14. Serve hot and enjoy.

Nutrition:

• Calories 363 | Total Fat 14. 2g | Saturated Fat 11g | Cholesterol 45mg | Sodium 91mg | Total Carbohydrate 43. 4g | Dietary Fiber 4. 6g | Total Sugars 3. 9g | Protein 12. 1g

Peanut Noodles Stir Fry

Preparation Time: 05 minutes | Cooking Time: 17 minutes | Servings: 2

Ingredients:

- ½ teaspoon ginger powder
- ¼ cup natural peanut butter
- ¼ cup hoisin sauce
- 1 cup hot water
- ¼ teaspoon sriracha hot sauce
- 1 tablespoon vegetable oil
- ½ teaspoon garlic powder
- 1 cup frozen stir fry vegetables
- 2 oz. soba noodles
- 2 sliced leek, optional

Directions:

1. Prepare the sauce first.
2. Add ginger powder into a bowl.
3. Add the peanut butter, hoisin sauce, sriracha hot sauce, and ¼ cup of hot water.
4. Stir or whisk until smooth.

5. Set the sauce aside until it is needed.

6. Set the Pressure pot to Sauté.

7. Add the vegetable oil and allow it to sizzle.

8. Add garlic powder and ginger powder and cook for 2 minutes.

9. Add the bag of frozen vegetables and cook for 5 minutes.

10. Add the remaining water and soba noodles.

11. Lock the lid and make sure the vent is closed.

12. Set Pressure pot to Manual or Pressure Cook on High Pressure for 10 minutes.

13. When cooking time ends, release pressure and wait for steam to completely stop before opening the lid.

14. Stir until everything is combined and coated with sauce.

15. Garnish with sliced leek if desired.

Nutrition:

Calories 501 | Total Fat 24. 4g | Saturated Fat 4. 6g | Cholesterol 1mg | Sodium 788mg | Total Carbohydrate 58. 1g | Dietary Fiber 6g | Total Sugars 15. 8g | Protein 17. 3g

Cauliflower Shells Cheese

Preparation Time: 05 minutes | Cooking Time: 15 minutes | Servings: 2

Ingredients:

- 4 oz. macaroni
- 1 cup vegetable broth
- ½ cup cauliflower florets
- 1/2 small onion
- 1 1/2 tablespoons butter
- 1 1/2 tablespoons coconut flour
- 1 1/2 cups coconut milk
- 1 cup sharp cheddar, shredded
- Salt and pepper to taste

Directions:

1. Set the Pressure pot to Sauté, add the coconut flour, butter, and onion.
2. The flour and butter will form a paste, whisk for 1-2 minutes more taking care not to let it scorch.

3. This slightly cooks the flour preventing the cheese sauce from having an overly strong flour flavor or paste-like flavor.
4. Whisk the milk into the roux until no lumps remain.
5. Add some freshly cracked pepper to the sauce.
6. Bring the mixture up to a simmer, stirring often.
7. Set aside.
8. Add macaroni and vegetable broth into Pressure pot.
9. Lock the lid and make sure the vent is closed.
10. Add cauliflower and set Pressure pot to Manual or Pressure Cook on High Pressure for 10 minutes.
11. When cooking time ends, release pressure and wait for steam to completely stop before opening the lid.
12. Add cheddar and stir sauce mix well with macaroni.

Nutrition:

Calories 643 | Total Fat 53. 6g | Saturated Fat 42. 1g | Cholesterol 75mg | Sodium 443mg | Total Carbohydrate 26. 2g | Dietary Fiber 6. 6g | Total Sugars 6. 2g | Protein 18. 4g

Lemon Mozzarella Pasta

Preparation Time: 05 minutes | Cooking Time: 10 minutes | Servings: 2

Ingredients:

- 4 oz. macaroni
- ¼ cup peas
- ½ cup mozzarella cheese
- ½ tablespoon olive oil
- 1 lemon
- Salt and pepper

Directions:

1. Set Pressure pot to Sauté.
2. Add the olive oil and allow it to sizzle.
3. Add macaroni, peas, lemon, salt, and pepper.
4. Lock the lid and make sure the vent is closed.
5. Set Pressure pot to Manual or Pressure Cook on High Pressure for 10 minutes.
6. When cooking time ends, release pressure and wait for steam to completely stop before opening the lid.

7. Add mozzarella cheese and Stir until everything is combined and coated with sauce.
8. Enjoy.

Nutrition:

Calories 273 | Total Fat 5. 9g | Saturated Fat 1. 3g | Cholesterol 4mg | Sodium 44mg | Total Carbohydrate 46. 6g | Dietary Fiber 3. 7g | Total Sugars 2. 8g | Protein 10. 3g

Kale Lasagna Roll-Ups

Preparation Time: 10 minutes | Cooking Time: 15 minutes | Servings: 2

Ingredients:

- ½ cup Lasagna noodles
- ½ cup goat cheese
- ½ cup mozzarella, shredded
- 1 large egg
- ¼ cup kale
- ½ cup marinara sauce
- Salt and pepper to taste
- Enough water

Directions:

1. Set Pressure pot to Sauté.
2. Add the kale with goat cheese, mozzarella, egg, pepper, and salt.
3. Stir regularly.
4. Add marinara sauce, water, noodles.
5. Mix well.
6. Stir to make sure noodles are covered with the liquid.

7. Lock the lid and make sure the vent is closed.

8. Set Pressure pot to Manual or Pressure Cook on High Pressure for 15 minutes.

9. When cooking time ends, release pressure and wait for steam to completely stop before opening the lid.

10. If you would like to sprinkle a bit on top of the Lasagna when you serve it.

Nutrition:

Calories 343 | Total Fat 23. 6g | Saturated Fat 22. 1g | Cholesterol 17. 5mg | Sodium 243mg | Total Carbohydrate 16. 2g | Dietary Fiber 3. 6g | Total Sugars 2. 2g | Protein 16. 4g

Zucchini Noodles

Preparation Time: 10 minutes | Cooking Time: 15 minutes | Servings: 2

Ingredients:

- 2 zucchini, peeled
- Marinara sauce of your choice
- Any other seasonings you wish to use

Directions:

• Peel & spiralizer your zucchini into noodles.

1. Add some of your favorite sauce to Pressure pot, hit —Sauté‖ and —Adjust‖ so it's on the—More‖ or —High‖ setting.
2. Once the sauce is bubbling, add the noodles to the pot, toss them in the sauce, and allow them to heat up and soften for a few minutes for about 2-5 minutes.
3. Serve in bowls and top with some grated parmesan, if desired.
4. Enjoy!

Nutrition:

Calories 86 | Total Fat 2g | Saturated Fat 0. 5g | Cholesterol 1mg | Sodium 276mg | Total Carbohydrate 15. 2g | Dietary Fiber 3. 8g | Total Sugars 8. 9g | Protein 3. 5g

Lemon Parsley Pasta

Preparation Time: 10 minutes | Cooking Time: 15 minutes | Servings: 2

Ingredients:

- 1 cup ziti pasta
- ½ cup fresh parsley, finely chopped
- 1 lemon zest
- 1 teaspoon garlic powder
- 1 1/2 tablespoon coconut oil
- ½ tablespoon butter
- 2 tablespoon parmesan cheese
- Salt and fresh black pepper
- Enough water

Directions:

1. Add butter to the Pressure pot, hit —Sauté‖ and once the butter is melted and sizzled, Add parsley, lemon zest, garlic powder, coconut oil, salt, and black pepper.
2. Lock the lid and make sure the vent is closed.
3. Add water and ziti pasta. Set Pressure pot to Manual or Pressure Cook on High PRESSURE for 10 minutes.

4. When cooking time ends, release pressure and wait for steam to completely stop before opening the lid.
5. Stir in cheese.
6. Serve and enjoy.

Nutrition:

Calories 377 | Total Fat 17. 4g | Saturated Fat 11. 9g | Cholesterol 74mg | Sodium 306mg | Total Carbohydrate 40. 7g | Dietary Fiber 1. 5g | Total Sugars 1. 2g | Protein 17. 3g

Creamy Tofu Marsala Pasta

Preparation Time: 10 minutes | Cooking Time: 15 minutes | Servings: 2

Ingredients:

- ¼ cup butter
- 1 tablespoon coconut oil
- 1 small onion, diced
- 2 cup mushrooms, sliced
- ½ cup tofu, diced into chunks
- ½ teaspoon garlic powder
- 1 1/2 cups of vegetable broth
- 1 cup of white wine
- ½ cup sun-dried tomatoes
- 1 cup fusilli
- 1/4 cup coconut cream
- ½ cup grated goat cheese

Directions:

1. Add the butter to the Pressure pot.
2. Hit —Sautél.
3. Add the onion and mushrooms and cook for 3-5 minutes, until the mushrooms have softened and browned a bit.

4. Then, add the tofu and the coconut oil from the sun-dried tomatoes and cook for another 2-3 minutes until the tofu is slightly white.

5. Toss in the garlic powder and cook for 1 more minute and then add in the white wine and let it simmer for 1 minute more.

6. Add in the vegetable broth and stir together well.

7. Pour in the fusilli so it's laying on top of the broth, gently smoothing and pushing it down with a spatula so it's submerged, but do not stir it with the rest of the broth.

8. Secure the lid and hit —Manual‖ or —Pressure Cook‖ High Pressure for 6 minutes.

9. Quick- release when done and give it all a good stir.

10. Stir in the coconut cream and goat cheese.

11. Let it sit for about 5 minutes, stirring occasionally and it will thicken up into an incredible sauce, coating all the pasta perfectly.

12. Transfer to a serving bowl, plate it up, and sprinkle any extra goat cheese if desired.

13. Enjoy!

Nutrition:

Calories 510 | Total Fat 20. 6g | Saturated Fat 14. 8g | Cholesterol 7mg | Sodium 432mg | Total Carbohydrate 45. 9g | Dietary Fiber 4. 8g | Total Sugars 7. 8g | Protein 19. 1g

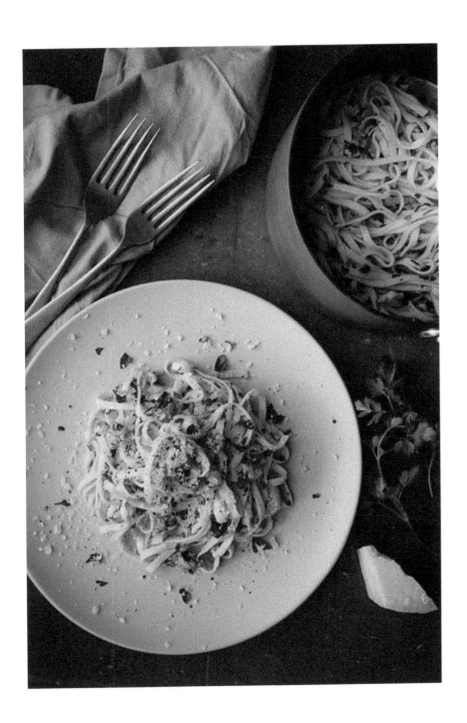

Lightning Source UK Ltd.
Milton Keynes UK
UKHW020654100621
385265UK00005B/143